HEAL YOURSELF
of
HERPES
❈
NATURALLY!

A Complete Guide for
Natural Cure!

Richard Teddy Frank

Text copyright © 2015 David Morgan

ALL RIGHTS RESERVED. No part of this publication may be reproduced or transmitted in any form or by any means, electronic or mechanical, including photocopying, recording, or any other information storage and retrieval system, without the written permission of the author.

Edition: 4

ISBN-13: 978-1537764139

ISBN-10: 1537764136

Printers CreateSpace

CreateSpace is authorized to distribute this version of the book to other platforms. The copyright of the book vests with the publisher David Morgan, WA.

Published in the United States of America

Printed in the United States of America

Disclaimer:

The author, editor and publisher are not responsible for errors and omissions or for any consequences from application of the information in this book and we make no warranty, express or implied, with respect to the contents of this publication.

The patients are advised to consult with their physicians before undertaking self-treatment.

The self-treatment mentioned herein should NOT be done in winter.

♣

Dedicated to the love of my life.....

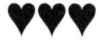

TABLE OF CONTENTS

Preface

Chapter 1: What Exactly Are You Going To Do?

Chapter 2: What Does My Plan Involve?

Chapter 3: Things To Avoid Or Reduce During This 52-Days Of Treatment

Chapter 4: Things To Do EVERY SINGLE DAY During This 52-Days Of Treatment

Chapter 5: Detoxification- Its Necessity And Types Of Simple Detox Procedures We Are Going To Use.

Chapter 6: Getting More Nutrients Delivered Into Your System- Diet & Supplements

Chapter 7: Fasting.

Chapter 8: Essential Activities for Raising The Immunity Level

Chapter 9: Your Main Detoxifier, Medicine & Topical Application.

Chapter 10: Honey for Herpes!

Chapter: 11 Other Natural Supplementary Cures for Herpes.

Chapter 12: Before Starting Treatment: Disinfection & Sterilization.

Chapter 13: Topical Application & Personal Hygiene: Do's and Don'ts

Chapter 14: Breathing Techniques (BT)

Chapter 15: Olives & Herpes!

Chapter 16: Food High In Antioxidants:

Chapter 17: Few Ayurveda Medicines To Stock Up.

Chapter 18: How to stop diarrhea naturally?

Chapter 19: Chart For Days 1-7

Chapter 20: Chart For Days 8-14

Chapter 21: Chart For Days 15-21

Chapter 22: Chart For Days 22-28

Chapter 23: Chart For Days 29-35

Chapter 24: Chart For Days 36-42

Chapter 25: Chart For Days 43-49

Chapter 26: Chart For Days 50, 51 and 52.

Before We Part

About the author

Introduction

Dear Reader,

You might have come across various articles, blogposts and books on Herpes. I have seen books that 'dedicate' the initial chapters to educate the reader on what Herpes is, and its types, causes and symptoms before they get to the cure. Sadly some authors choose to give their books with cure and without cure, where the book with cure is priced higher than the one without the 'secret' cure.

This book is not going to talk about what Herpes is. It will not even discuss about the types of Herpes nor describe anything related to what causes Herpes. There won't be any discussion about what the symptoms are. We won't be talking about the other sexually transmitted diseases either. Such information is available all over the web.

By now, you would know, what Herpes is, how it spreads and how to protect yourself (if not, surf the internet and educate yourself). I won't be repeating what you can find elsewhere. Filling the pages with redundant, vague, ambiguous information is not my kind of eBook.

This book is about THE CURE!

This book talks about THE SOLUTION!

There is NO magic pill.

It involves a lot of herbal, natural, Ayurvedic medicine and a series of simple activities like exercises, massages, breathing techniques, etc. We are going to talk about the solution for herpes which incidentally happens to be a solution for many other sexually transmitted diseases too (with slight modifications) and in the course of the self-treatment you will be on the road to wellness.

Chapter 1: What Exactly Are You Going To Do?

I want to dedicate this chapter to educate you of the importance of the things coming up in the following chapters. Please read this chapter carefully to avoid making any mistakes.

Keep in mind the following:

1) I am NOT selling you any product here (or anywhere for that matter). I do not have a website and will not be having any until late 2016.

2) I am NOT going to ask you to sign up with me for getting prescriptions and tailor-made charts.

3) I am going to show you how to get cured of Herpes using the INEXPENSIVE things you find in your garden, kitchen, supermarket and any store that sells the Indian medicines I suggest in this book.

You have to undergo several kinds of detoxification processes to remove the toxins, infections and parasites which are destroying your immunity. Do not worry about your condition even if it seems hopeless. Herpes affects anywhere and everywhere. It is a well-known fact that Herpes affects even the brain and compromises the nervous system.

BUT THEN...

YOU CAN BE CURED!

YOU WILL BE CURED!

By following what I say here you will be systematically removing the toxins, infections of all sorts (viral, bacterial and fungal) and the parasites including the intestinal worms, if any.

Stay tuned with me, take notes of what you read, make charts, stick it on the wall and stick to your charts.

Chapter 2: What Does My Plan Involve?

This is merely an overview of the upcoming chapters! Stay tuned with me and I assure you that you will become healthier than ever.

- Things You Must Avoid/Reduce During This 52-Days of Self-Treatment.

- Things To Do EVERYDAY During This 52-Days Of Treatment

- Detoxification & Its Necessity. Types of Simple Detox Procedures We Are Going To Use.

- Getting More Nutrients Delivered Into Your System To Fight Herpes- Diet, Supplements (only if you are too weak)

- Fasting.

- Activities Essential for Raising The Immunity Level For The Medicine To Work.

- The Treatment for Herpes Sores & Topical Applications.

- The Herbal Medicines Which Must Be Used In Combination

Chapter 3: Things To Avoid Or Reduce

with Detox, Diet and Exercise that I prescribe n this book.

- Chart for Days 1–7
- Chart for Days 8–14
- Chart for Days 15–21
- Chart for Days 22–28
- Chart for Days 29–35
- Chart for Days 36–42
- Chart for Days 43–49
- Chart for the 50th, 51st and 52nd days

You will start feeling a whole lot better by Week 3! DON'T TRUST THAT temporary feeling and stop the treatment abruptly! It's temporary and misleading. You must continue until the 52nd day and follow this regime to become completely immune to the Herpes virus and get back to normal living.

I repeat, DO NOT abandon this schedule and discipline the moment you feel better but finish the 52 days course of self-treatment entirely and follow my instructions carefully. You will be completely cured.

Much care has been taken to reduce the size of this eBook so that it doesn't discourage the readers from completing it. I have tried my best to incorporate all the necessary details without putting a burden on the readers in terms of volume.

Chapter 3: Things To Avoid Or Reduce During This 52-Days Of Treatment

For the medicines and herbs to work effectively, or let's say for the medicines and herbs to work at all, you must start doing a couple of things, must reduce certain things and stay away from few others.

THINGS TO BE AVOIDED:

- Alcohol
- Drugs

- Smoking
- Caffeine- coffee, tea & green tea
- Pork
- Chicken and eggs (Organic chicken and eggs can be consumed in moderation in the last 3 weeks of treatment. Moderation means 2 small pieces of organic chicken once in a week and 2 organic eggs a week.)
- High caloric food
- Fatty food
- White flour
- Sugar
- Processed food

- Spicy food (to avoid diarrhea from an irritated stomach and colon)

- Pornography (For 2 reasons, one being the chemical reaction in the brain which affects the treatment and the other being the negative impact on the pre-frontal cortex which will interfere with treatment in terms of disrupted diet and sleep discipline)

- Staying late at night

- Poor nutrition

- Getting exhausted by working hard or partying hard or simply getting exhausted over anything.

Kindly note that, Green Tea is good for health and is loaded with anti-oxidants. Green Tea by itself, aids in removing toxins from our system. Still I have added Green Tea to the list of things to be avoided for the reason that Green Tea will interfere with the other herbal medicines. After the completion of 52 days of treatment you can start having your green tea. If it's not your habit to have Green Tea, better start making it one.

THINGS TO BE REDUCED:

Avoid sexual intercourse during the first 5 weeks of treatment. It will place additional burden on your system when a major cleansing is underway. From week 6 you can start being sexually active but not every day. Twice in a week would be the limit unless you want to spend more time in the toilet and more money on toilet tissues. It will affect your bowel movements and weaken your system. Do it in moderation, and only if necessary and desired. It would be better if you can completely stay away from it until 52 days of self-treatment is over.

Chapter 4: Things To Do EVERY SINGLE DAY During This 52-Days Of Treatment

So, what are you going to do in these 52 days of treatment? In the previous chapter you read about things that should be reduced and avoided. This chapter describes things you will be doing in order to fight this battle against Herpes.

No need to worry that it might be something you might fail to comprehend. It is all easy. Since it is too easy, you might be tempted to ignore them to your own peril.

Medicines and herbs DO NOT WORK unless your body is prepared to receive it.

By following what I advise here, you wouldn't be losing anything of any value. On the other hand you will become physically, emotionally and mentally fit, lose weight, get lustrous hair, glowing skin, regulated hormones, remove toxins, kill infections, get rid of parasites, come out of low self-esteem and depression, improve metabolism.... list is endless.

This Must Form Part of Everyday Routine:

1) Start your day early

2) Start it with breathing exercises

3) Have a light detox juice

4) Start moving within an hour of waking up. Take a brisk walk. If you are

used to jogging and running then go ahead and do that. People who have been lethargic for a while can start with a casual stroll of 20 minutes and increase it by few minutes every day.

5) Get morning sunlight for 30-45 minutes as you walk or jog. Or in the evening if you cannot make it in the morning. But keep in mind that doing it in the morning is better.

6) Meditation in the mornings or evenings or both for raising your immunity (you heard it right) and to keep at bay the secretion of those harmful hormones that makes you age faster which also triggers the outbreaks. Anyone who has read the book The Anti-Aging Zone by Dr. Barry Sears would remember reading about how meditation helping in reducing the

secretion of harmful brain chemicals which makes you age faster.

7) Eat breakfast within two hours of waking up (consisting of what is prescribed in the relevant chapter).

8) Getting a (non-sexual) body massage every week (ONLY on days prescribed in the final charts).

9) Get your medicines well in advance in order to avoid interruption in the course. I don't sell any medicines and this eBook is not written for promoting any particular brand here. Those harmless Ayurveda medicines I suggest are cheap and are available almost anywhere. Or you can place orders on any online store of your choice. Please make sure you stock up the medicines you need before you embark on your self-treatment.

10) In the same way, buy the groceries in advance to avoid eating junk, and crap that will ruin your chances of getting cured.

11) Stay organized. Stress destroys your immunity. Stay calm.

Chapter 5: Detoxification- Its Necessity And Types Of Simple Detox Procedures We Are Going To Use.

Why is Detoxification necessary? Simple! Health starts in the gut! The nutrients are mainly absorbed in the small intestines and large intestines after which it is delivered to various parts of the body through the circulatory system. The medicines will not work effectively when the bowels are clogged with yucky decaying stools which are releasing toxins and/or when there are parasites in the intestines which are sucking the blood and nutrients while releasing waste and toxins in your system (which complicates health even more badly than Herpes).

Traditionally, the Indians cleansed their intestines by oral administration of freshly ground Neem paste every fortnight.

GENERAL BENEFITS OF DETOXIFICATION

-Strengthen the peristaltic muscular action of the small and large intestines

-Removes toxins

-Removes old dried up feces

-Removes parasites

-The presence of parasites accelerates ageing due to the toxins they release.

Ageing process is slowed down by detoxification.

SPECIAL BENEFITS OF DETOXIFICATION FOR HERPES PATIENTS!

1. Better absorption of nutrients will help the patient to continue the self-treatment without interruption.

2. The medicine will work effectively on a clean gut. A clogged up gut makes any kind of healing impossible.

3. Healing process is hastened

Most of detoxification processes I mention here are simple and easy. In Ayurveda (not the fake version of Ayurveda out there), the patients are treated for chronic diseases only after making them undergo detoxification process for few days before the main medicine is internally administered to the patient. Reason behind this is simple: Medicines DO NOT WORK well if your body has toxins and parasites.

Most diseases get cured just by the preparatory medicines (detox medicines) given for detoxification. Not every Ayurveda "doctor" is really an expert in Ayurveda. What I suggest here is not just extracts from Ayurveda books compiled by ancient Indian kings. But I have included a variety of alternate treatments that will work in a combination suited for this modern Western world.

We will have Days 1-5 exclusively for "light detox" and for strengthening your immune system to withstand the slightly heavy detox that comes in the weekend, viz., Days 6 and 7. Thus every weekend we will have a slightly heavy detox which is nothing to worry about. It is absolutely necessary for the medicines to work.

TYPES OF DETOXIFICATION METHODS WE WILL BE USING:

This will sound simple but when used in the right combination and at right intervals as I prescribe, you will find yourself becoming more healthy and vibrant. Your herpes will fade away. Don't panic at the list.

1 Main Detox: Will be dealt with in the relevant chapter

2 Body Massages: It is very essential that you get a decent non-sexual body massage from a professional (not erotic massages in parlors) every week. Don't run to China Town. Get it done by a Therapist

with the necessary professional qualification and training in Reflexology and Other Alternate Medicines.

Body massage helps in draining unwanted fluids. The Herpes virus affects your Lymph nodes too. These body massages will promote better health of body and mind. It relieves stress and improves blood circulation. Your skin, muscles, connecting tissues, tendons, nerves, bones, internal and external organs are greatly benefited by body massages.

Remember to fix appointments beforehand. Or you can ask your partner or a good friend to learn the same techniques from a good book. Combine Reflexology with massage. Doing reflexology after the massage is advisable.

3 Oil Pulling: It removes toxins from your body.

4. Detox drinks: To be taken in the morning at empty stomach. Lemon in warm water, honey in warm water, carrot-beet-apple-juice (in the ratio of 1:0.5:1 with a teaspoon of honey), papaya-sunflower seed smoothie, etc.

5. Few harmless Ayurveda and Siddha medicines for detoxification as dealt with in the relevant chapter.

Chapter 6: Getting More Nutrients Delivered Into Your System- Diet & Supplements

Before you start this treatment, you might prefer to undergo a basic checkup to ascertain how well you are doing before the treatment. Have blood tests done to assess if you have any deficiencies. If you think that you cannot afford those tests, don't worry. I will be prescribing few medicines and foods which are inexpensive (unless you prefer organic) and those medicines and foods will help you to come out of deficiencies too.

Chapter 7: Fasting.

Fasting is an essential prerequisite to make Ayurveda and Herbal medicines work. It hastens the healing procedure and makes your detoxification successful. In this self-treatment you will be fasting until noon once in a week before the main Detox (scheduled on the 6th and 7th days respectively).

It is highly recommended that the patient fasts before the Main Detox (Neem Detox) in order to avoid all the mess. Foods and beverages will make it quite difficult and extremely uncomfortable for the patient as Neem detox tends to cause vomiting/nausea. Passing stools frequently during neem detox is not uncommon.

So avoid eating and drinking anything on the day of Neem Detox. Besides it reduces the effectiveness of the treatment and delays the results. If you follow what is laid out for you here, you will be a changed person on the 52nd day.

Chapter 8: Essential Activities for Raising The Immunity Level

For the medicine to work effectively, the immunity ought to be boosted. In this chapter we will discuss few activities that help to raise the immunity level. Please don't ignore this if you want the medicine to work.

For the medicine to work effectively, the immunity ought to be boosted. In this chapter we will discuss few activities that help to raise the immunity level. Please don't ignore this if you want the medicine to work.

1) DEEP BREATHING: Start with the Breathing Exercise mentioned in this book or any Breathing Exercise you know of. Throughout the day, practice deep breathing for few minutes until it becomes a habit.

2) EXERCISE: Physical Exercises every day -in the mornings and evenings. Just light exercises or even walking is enough. Keep moving.

3) SOCIALIZE: Go out and mingle. Hang out with family and friends. By hanging out, I don't mean sitting in front of TV or playing video games. And I don't suggest hanging out in pubs/clubs/bars. Hang out in open places with plenty of fresh air and PLAY. That's the way to heal.

Humans are not designed to stay put in one place for long periods of time. Keep moving. Stay active.

4) AVOID NOISE: Noise interrupts, disrupts, delays and messes up with healing. Unwanted sounds and intrusive noises triggers many physical responses like speeding heartbeat, muscle tension, heart troubles, immunity decline etc. besides affecting blood pressure, cholesterol and digestion. This is caused by noise activating excessive secretion of adrenaline. Loud music is detrimental to health even in normal people.

5) STAY POSITIVE: Many researches have confirmed the contention of how people who are negative, moody, angry, bitter, stress-prone or pessimistic tend to be more susceptible to have a weakened immune system.

6) STAY TUNED WITH YOUR ANIMAL SELF: Wake up before dawn and stay active. Use natural light whenever possible. In the evenings try to stay in the dark as much as possible. Sleep early. SWITCH OFF the light in your bedroom and sleep in the dark.

7) ENGAGE IN NERDY HOBBIES: Studies indicate that the games or activities which help you to use your intellectual functions and boosts immunity. So engage in such activities which helps you think, analyze and act.

8) LISTEN TO SOOTHING MUSIC: It boosts your immunity, calms your nerves and relaxes your tensed up muscles.

9) EAT HEALTHY: You are what you eat. Eat 5 short meals throughout the day.

And finish off a hearty breakfast within at least 90 minutes of waking up.

Chapter 9: Your Main Detoxifier, Medicine & Topical Application.

NEEM!

What is Neem? I would like to give a brief introduction about this wonderful gift from God. The binomial name of Neem is Azadirachta Indica. It is also known as Neem, Nimtree, and Indian Lilac. A native to India and the Indian subcontinent, this tree is THE KING of Indian Medicine. Even the uneducated folks in India will surprise you by casually suggesting a handful of herbal treatment methods/procedures involving Neem which gives immediate relief and permanent cure.

Though this tree is native to Indian Subcontinent including Nepal, Pakistan, Bangladesh and Sri Lanka, it was introduced in many other countries. Few countries where the Neem tree is naturalized are Northern Australia, South & Central America, the Caribbean, Puerto Rico and few others. Unfortunately North America does not have this tree but the leaves, powder, capsules and oil can be obtained it from other places.

How can it be used?

It can be used in the following forms:

-Neem Oil

Neem Decoction

–Neem Paste made from fresh/dry leaves (whole leaves or powdered leaves).

If fresh Neem leaves are available in your country please use the freshly ground Neem Paste whenever possible. Others can get the dry leaves or powder from herbal stores or order it online. It is dust cheap.

Neem!! This is the main detox as well the main medicine, and also the effective topical application for Herpes sores & blisters, warts and all sexually transmitted diseases.

Now you have two options:

Option 1: *Believe You Are Smart:*

On glancing through this chapter and finding out that Neem is the main solution, some of the readers will ignore all that I say in the following chapters of this eBook and focus on just Neem. I assure you that they will not have desired results. Some of them will give up after a few unsuccessful attempts in getting cured. That's what people get on focusing on just Neem.

Reason being this: the weakened immune system will not withstand the fatigue from vomiting and diarrhea which will be so intense enough to discourage anyone from trying it again despite any temporary relief experienced. Besides, treating with Neem involves a strict-systematic procedure. I have done my best to chart it out in such a way that it will be helpful for anyone (like in ANYONE). If you proceed without knowledge about how to use but just mere information that Neem will help you, you will suffer and give up. Finish reading the book completely and understand how it works.

Option 2: *Be Smart:*

Listen to what I have said here. Follow the various steps, use neem & other medicines as prescribed, and in the prescribed intervals, and get cured. I have listed out what should form part of your diet and the exercises, massages, medicines, herbs, etc. you need, so that your system will be strengthened enough to withstand the strong detox of Neem.

---

1) NEEM FOR DETOX:

Detox should be started on empty stomach.

-Neem leaves powder (dried) made into a decoction.

OR

- Fresh neem leaves (paste)

OR

- Neem Oil

2) NEEM AS MEDICINE:

Neem Capsules or Neem Oil or Fresh Neem Paste to be taken as prescribed (in the relevant chapters).

3) NEEM AS EXTERNAL APPLIACTION:

Neem paste (dried or fresh) or Neem oil should be applied on the sores and blisters. I don't suggest neem cream unless it is organic and doesn't have any preservatives. Since there is no such thing as a cream without any preservatives, I do not suggest creams except where you can't find anything natural. Get the neem powder or leaves or oil and use it for better results.

Chapter 10: Honey for Herpes!

Many researches have proved that Honey is more effective than Acyclovir. Honey has always been the best in healing the wounds naturally and also aids in fighting infections. Why not use this gift from God to get back your lost health and vitality?

What Honey To Use? Avoid using the processed honey. Spend few more bucks and buy a good raw kind. Not all kinds of honey are safe to use on open sores. I suggest Manuka Honey made from Manuka bushes in New Zealand. It has been proven that Manuka Honey is superior in quality than all its counterparts and is gifted with a high level of healing properties. Or you can opt for some raw organic honey. Anything processed is a big NO.

1) Honey As Topical Application:

- Pour the required quantity of honey into the little brass bowl or disposable cup. Keep it aside for an hour before using if you use brass bowls.

- Using cotton swabs or balls, apply the honey on your sores.

- To avoid contamination, NEVER keep your honey bottle near you, when you are applying honey on sores.

- Apply 5-7 times a day.

2) Add Honey To Your Detox Drinks & Immunity Boosting Drinks:

Wherever I mention about adding honey to your detox drinks or immunity-boosting juices and smoothies add only organic honey of ANY brand you prefer.

Chapter: 11 Other Natural Supplementary Cures for Herpes.

This chapter is dedicated for the other natural cures which should be alternated during the course of treatment. Besides Neem and Honey, there are few other remedies that have proved to be effective in relieving the outbreaks of herpes infections:

1) Lysine:

Lysine, an essential amino acid is essential for healing yourself of Herpes. Long term usage of drugs containing Lysine will impair your immune system. Get it NATURALLY from food. The food which are the harmless sources of Lysine are given below:

- Chicken
- Beef
- Yeast
- Milk
- Eggs
- Beans
- Cheese.
- Wheat grass
- Barley grass

2) Other Effective Medicines (Topical Applications) for Herpes are:

- Sage

- Rhubarb

- Oregano oil

- Elderberry

- Olive leaf extracts

- Aloe Vera

- Lemon Balm (Melissa officinalis)

- Garlic

- Colostrum

- Tea Tree Oil

- Senna

NOTE: Stay away from Licorice root as prolonged usage will affect your health if used for prolonged period. And it will definitely affect your health as you will be using it for a prolonged period as it would bring a neither a permanent cure nor an immediate cure. It offers temporary relief and long-term irreversible damage. Instead follow the things mentioned here and be cured of this disease.

Chapter 12: Before Starting Treatment: Disinfection & Sterilization.

Before and during the treatment (and preferably after the treatment), carry out basic disinfection and sterilization in the following places and in the following ways.

-Residence including the walls, floor, couches & other furniture.

-Doormats, rugs, curtains and fabric of all kinds.

-All the clothes and accessories (including footwear), pillow covers, sheets and all materials of fabric, in the residence, car, and office should be washed & disinfected.

-Cars and other vehicles

-Office chair (use disinfectant spray)

-Pet houses, pet clothing, bed and stuff

REMEMBER THIS:

-Change the sheets everyday

-Bathe everyday

-Wear clean cotton clothes

-Avoid tight undergarments. ONLY 100% pure COTTON undergarments are suggested

-Clean the couches and other furniture everyday

Chapter 13: Topical Application & Personal Hygiene: Do's and Don'ts

Caution must be exercised in personal hygiene. The patient should bathe everyday (twice a day is even better) despite the weather conditions and wear clean cotton clothes only.

Next, let us see the manner of applying the topical application.

1) First clean the sores/blisters with gentle soap or cleanser and warm water. To cleanse it effectively, boil the water, keep

aside and use the same when it becomes warm.

2) If you can afford small brass bowls, keep the clean drinking water in the brass bowls overnight and use it for cleaning the sores.

3) Clean and dry a little brass bowl/disposable cup dedicated for mixing Herpes topical application herbs and oils.

4) Add the required quantity of ingredients topical application ingredients in the little brass bowl/disposable cup.

5) Using cotton balls/swabs, to apply on your sores. Dip a new cotton ball to apply medicine on the new sets of sores. Never dip a used cotton ball/swab into the medicine directly.

6) Keep an empty disposable cup to put the dirty cotton balls/swabs, bandages, etc.

7) To avoid contamination, NEVER keep the container/bottles (in which the ingredients are stored) near you, when you are applying medicines on sores.

8) Those who cannot afford a brass bowl due to its cost or due to the washing requirement, kindly use a disposable cup each time.

9) Use a new disposable cup each time or wash your brass bowl each time and dry it.

Any lazy person who uses the dirty bowl again is NOT going to recover. Same applies for those stingy about using new disposable cups.

Note: I suggested Brass bowl as brass had the inherent ability to kill many kinds of micro-organisms including bacteria, virus, algae, spores, fungi, moulds, etc. If you can afford huge brass pots/vessels, try to store water overnight and use the water for bathing. If silver coin(s) or gold coin(s) can be afforded, please invest in it. Leave the coin(s) in the water used for cleaning the sores or the water used for bathing to fasten the healing process.

Let us see some of the ways to soothe the outbreaks.

1) Epsom Salt

Epsom salt is used to hasten the healing of blisters of all sorts. It has been proven to be helpful in dealing with blisters from herpes outbreaks. It works by drying up the blisters faster and by preventing further infection. The Epsom salt relieves the pain of outbreaks and speeds up the healing time. In many cases it has been proven to relieve itching.

<u>How to use Epsom Salt:</u>

Fill a bathtub with a hot of water, and add in a cup full of Epsom salt. Stir up the water. Soak in for 10-15 minutes for better results.

2) Lemon:

Lemon is one of the most popular and commonly used home remedies for herpes. Cut lemon pieces into halves and bandage it on the open area directly on the sores. You can keep it on the sores as long as you like and make sure to replace with another fresh lemon after 2 hours. Lemon is very effective during the start of herpes outbreak.

3) Witch Hazel:

This cream is effective in treating many skin disorders and infections. Apply twice in a day.

4) Cold Compress:

Ice cubes can be used to reduce the swelling and pain of the herpes outbreak. It is also effective in reducing the redness of the herpes outbreaks. Apply ice cube directly on the affected area. Or place them in a plastic bag and press against the affected area for 5 minutes.

5) Aloe Vera:

Consume fresh Aloe Vera pulp every morning. Apply the Aloe Vera pulp or gel on the skin.

6) Oils used for Topical Application:

-Neem Oil

-Castor Oil

-Jojoba Oil

-Tea Tree Oil

-Vitamin-E Oil

7) Olive Leaf Paste:

It is discussed in the relevant chapter.

8) Blow Dry:

After bathing or cleaning, always blow dry the genitals and other areas using hair dryer.

Make sure you apply few of these many times a day. Never use the same topical application for more than a week. Alternate between them regularly to prevent the virus from getting accustomed to it, and thereby, becoming ineffective. You will be using few (let's say 3 or 4 or 5) of the herbs/oils/pastes for topical application at a time and alternate every week to another set of herbs/oils/pastes).

Chapter 14: Breathing Techniques (BT)

We often hear about eating it right. I often wonder why people fail to give much thought for breathing it right. Breathing it right will increase the supply of oxygen to the brain, boost immunity and improve blood circulation. Thus helps in healing faster.

We have treated various patients with nothing but simple breathing techniques and herbal remedies. Not to mention that we have helped patients who were on the verge of getting a Bi-Polar or Schizophrenia relapse with just few hours of counseling where they were trained to do Mindful Breathing to get in touch with reality.

BT 1 To Be Done In The Morning On Waking Up.

1. Lie in your bed with eyes closed. (Preferably try to sleep alone until you get healed as quieter surroundings will aid in healing faster.)

2. Do not use pillow underneath the head. Make sure there are no pillows or sheets underneath you. Try to be on an EVEN surface.

3. Keep your palms on your chest.

4. Start taking deep breaths.

5. Do NOT hold your breath.

6. Just breathe in as long as you can. Long-deep- breath-.

7. Do NOT hold.

8. Breathe out slowly.

9. Repeat 16 times.

10. Slowly open your eyes and close it. Repeat 10 times.

11. Do NOT get up for 5 minutes as the increased supply of oxygen to the brain will cause some degree of buzzing in your head and make you feel uncomfortable if you get up right after the breathing technique.

12. Now turn to your left, lay on your right for a minute or two and get up slowly.

BT 2: To Be Done On Standing Up

1. On standing up after BT 1, proceed with BT 2.

2. Stand at ease with legs apart matching the shoulder width.

3. The spine should be straight

4. Head must be straight

5. Eyes must look straight

6. Butt in

7. Pelvis up

8. Chest out

9. Raise your hands slowly and bring to your sides (at shoulder). Stand with open arms for few minutes and take deep breaths.

10. Like a bird spreading its wings, open your arms as far as you can without strain. Inhale deeply while you are at spreading the wings posture.

11. Exhale slowly as you bring your hands to the front slowly. At this stage the palms will be facing and touching each other in front of you at the Solar Plexus level.

12. Repeat 10 times

13. Breathe in as you spreading wings

14. Breathe out as you bring it to the front with palms brushing each other.

15. Slowly and gradually raise the count to 25.

BT 3: To Be Done Before Going To Bed.

-Practice BT 1 before going to bed.

An additional 20-30 minutes of Yogasana, Tai-Chi and Qi-Gong will hasten the healing process. There are many good websites out there which contains excellent free material through which you can learn Yogasana, Tai-Chi and Qi-Gong.

Chapter 15: Olives & Herpes!

Olives, Olive Oil and Olive Leaf Extract contain medicinal properties. Include Olive Oil in your diet. And add olives to your diet. Olive Leaf Extract is most important of the three as it will kill almost all kinds of bacteria, virus, fungus and protozoa. In case of Herpes, it controls the growth and replication of the virus. It kills the virus infected cells.

1) OLIVE LEAVES EXTRACT CAPSULES:

Get an organic brand of the dosage around 750 mg. Follow the instructions on the leaflet. Overdosing is not common and many websites as well as doctors claim that it is not dangerous to consume over the prescribed dosages. But to be cautious always follow this: Too Much Of Anything Is Good For Nothing. Stick to the limits. If you take higher dosages, you are making the virus immune to it.

While consuming the tablets you will experience flu-like symptoms or diarrhea. No need to panic. It signals that the desired reaction has started and toxins are being removed. To flush it out, drink plenty of water. Sip your water. Do not gulp it down. Sip and drink a glass of water every waking hour.

2) TOPICAL APPLICATION:

If you can afford to get fresh olive leaves, grind them into a smooth paste and apply the same on your sores after washing the sores with warm water and a gentle soap or cleanser. Others who cannot find fresh olive leaves can use the dry olive leaves powder by making them into a paste together with necessary amount of Extra-Virgin Olive Oil. Wash it off after 2 hours.

3) DIET:

Add olives and olive oil to the diet. Make sure you have 2 teaspoons of organic Olive oil every day.

Chapter 16: Food High In Antioxidants:

Taking food high in anti-oxidants is essential for healing from any disease. Make sure you include at least 5 types of vegetables, 3 kinds of nuts and a huge tub of yogurt to your diet.

Some of the food high in anti-oxidants are: Leeks, onions, garlic, grapes, apricots, eggplant, berries, pumpkin, carrots, spinach, parsley, seafood, lean meat, offal, peppers, mangoes, milk, nuts, legumes, apples, leafy greens, cruciferous vegetables such as broccoli, cabbage, cauliflower, sesame seeds & other seeds, bran, corn, tomatoes, pink grapefruit, watermelon, thyme, oregano, whole grains, oranges and other citrus fruits, kiwi fruit, vegetable oils, avocados, etc.

The list is not an exhaustive list of food high in anti-oxidants. Kindly do your own research and add more items to your diet. Stay away from anything you are allergic to.

Chapter 17: Few Ayurveda Medicines To Stock Up.

Before starting the 52 days of treatment, kindly stock up on these Ayurveda medicines. Almost all these medicines contain self-generated alcohol which will not hinder the effectiveness of the treatment in any manner. Some of these medicines can be used even after the 52 weeks of treatment to maintain good health and to fight ageing. They are harmless medicines (mainly tonic) which can be consumed by anyone for improving immunity and strength, and for relieving fatigue.

The medicines suggested here will improve digestion which will lead to better absorption of nutrients. These medicines do NOT have any side-effects and there are normal people who take it regularly to improve and maintain health. The patient will be strengthened by these medicines in every possible way one can imagine- physical, mental and emotional.

All the systems, viz. Skeletal System, Muscular System, Cardiovascular System, Integumentary System, Urinary System, Endocrine System, Lymphatic System, Respiratory System, Excretory System, Reproductive System, Digestive System and Immune System, are taken care of by these medicines.

1) DASAMOOLARISHTAM:

- Dosage: 12-24 ml.

- One or two times a day

- After food.

- Add equal quantity of water

- Can be used for several months.

2) ASHWAGANDHARISHTA:

- Dosage: 12-24 ml.

- One or two times a day

- After food

- Add equal quantity of water to dilute

- Can be can be used for several months.

3) SARASWATARISHTA:

- Dosage: 12-24 ml.

- One or two times a day

- After food.

- Add equal quantity of water.

- Can be used for ONE month followed by a break of ONE month.

4) RASAYANAVARA:

- 12 ml after food

- Once in a week.

5) RAJODOSHAHARA:

- For MEN

- 12 ml after food

- On alternate days
- For 3 months.

6) SHUKRADOSHAHARA:

- For WOMEN
- 12 ml after food
- On alternate days
- For 3 months.

7) DRAKSHARISHTAM

- Dosage: 12-24 ml.
- One or two times a day
- After food.
- Add equal quantity of water

-Can be can be used for several months.

-Safe enough to be continued forever.

8) TRIPHALA CHOORAM (POWDER):

-Mix a tablespoon of this powder with warm water or organic (cow) milk every night before bedtime.

-Cleanses the colon.

-Cures constipation.

-Helps with bowel movements.

-Strengthens and revitalizes the digestive system.

-Aids in better absorption of food

–Anyone can use it and it can be used indefinitely.

9) SESAME OIL:

Swish around a teaspoon full of sesame oil for 5 minutes every morning before having your detox drink.

Chapter 18: How to Stop Diarrhea Naturally?

During the course of this treatment, if any of you experience pain in the stomach due to heat or suffer from diarrhea, follow this harmless remedy to stop the stomach ache or diarrhea.

-Take a cup of live yogurt

-Add 2 glasses of water

-Add a pinch of salt to it

-Drink slowly by sipping it

-Continue again after 40 minutes

–This can be used by anyone.

The diet during diarrhea must be rice with buttermilk (yogurt diluted in water). Rice must be well-cooked and smashed. After it becomes warm, add buttermilk.

Note that the term buttermilk used in this chapter is not the traditional buttermilk. When I say buttermilk, I mean the organic yogurt diluted in water. The diet during diarrhea must be rice with buttermilk (yogurt diluted in water). Rice must be well-cooked and smashed. After it becomes warm, add buttermilk.

Chapter 19: Chart For Days 1-7

Days: 1-5

-Start your day with the Breathing Techniques to be done on waking up.

-Meditate for 10-15 minutes.

-Do the Breathing Techniques to be done on standing up.

-Have FRESH Pomegranate juice without ice or sugar. Do not refrigerate. Have at room temperature.

-Have few strawberries or some soft fruit and a handful of almonds.

-Start moving. Go for a walk or do some mild exercises for at least 20 minutes.

-Get exposure to sunlight for 30 minutes.

-Have a breakfast high in protein, complex carbohydrates and fiber within 2 hours of waking up.

-Have a light nutritious meal with plenty of veggies and yogurt.

-Can have 2 freshly made pita bread or Indian bread or rice with vegetables for dinner.

-Apply the Neem oil or Neem paste all over the body and relax for an hour before washing off with a mild soap. If Neem powder or paste was used instead of oil, there is no need for soap. This ought to be done in the day time between 7am and 4 pm.

-Before going to bed have warm organic Milk with Triphala Powder if not allergic to dairy. Others can have Triphala powder in warm water.

-Mediate for 10-15 minutes.

-Do the Breathing Techniques to be done before going to bed.

Day: 6

-Start your day with the Breathing Techniques to be done on waking up.

-Meditate for 10-15 minutes.

-Do the Breathing Techniques to be done on standing up.

-Have FRESH Pomegranate juice without ice or sugar. Do not refrigerate. Have at room temperature.

-Fast until 3 pm

-During fasting the patient can have fresh juice of apple, pomegranate, grapes and watermelon once in an hour. Do not refrigerate the juice. Do not add ice or sugar. Make fresh juice right before drinking.

-At 3pm, have a very light nutritious meal with veggies and yogurt.

-Have a full body MASSAGE from your spouse or your therapist. Or have a self-massage done. And finish with a nice hot bath. Do not spend more than 20 minutes in the bath.

–Herbal wrap need not be done on the days of fasting.

–For dinner have 2 freshly made pita bread or Indian bread or rice with vegetables for dinner. This will be the only solid meal of the day and must be finished before 7 pm.

–Before going to bed have warm organic Milk with Triphala Powder if not allergic to dairy. Others can have Triphala powder in warm water.

–Mediate for 10-15 minutes.

–Do the Breathing Techniques to be done before going to bed.

Day 7

-Start your day early with the Breathing Techniques to be done on waking up.

-Meditate for 10-15 minutes.

-Do the Breathing Techniques to be done on standing up.

-Fast until afternoon. Stay indoors. Turn off TV, music and phones on this day.

-During fasting, drink cool water. Remember to never gulp down the water but sip and drink your water very slowly.

-Spread a cotton sheet on the floor and lie down on it. Keep your eyes closed and your mind clear. Try to have happy, peaceful, positive thoughts.

-If you feel too tired to fast with just water, you can have a glass of pomegranate

juice or honey in warm water once in an hour to keep up your energy levels. This can be taken until 11 am. Stop all kinds of juices at 11 am. A glass of water an hour is mandatory.

-Around 1 pm, consume 3 tablespoons full of Neem oil. Drink a glass of hot water. Lie down flat on your back. Breathe deeply and slowly.

-The detox begins in 2 hours. The patient will feel nauseous. Vomiting and loose stools are normal part of detox. There is nothing to worry.

-Try to have Oral Rehydration Salts (ORS) every 30 minutes. You can buy a good brand of Oral Rehydration Salts from the pharmacist and mix with water instead of buying the ORS in drink form (to avoid the preservatives). Or mix 3 pinches of

sugar with 3 pinches of salt in a glass of water to make your homemade rehydration drink.

-After every single vomiting or toilet session, have few sips of your rehydration drink.

-If you don't start vomiting or pass loose stools or experience nausea within 90 minutes of having the Neem Oil, try to take another dose of 3 Tablespoons full of Neem Oil.

-Once it is all over, have a warm bath. Do not stay in the bath for more than 10 minutes.

-Have 2 freshly made pita bread or Indian bread or rice with vegetables for dinner.

-Before going to bed have warm organic Milk with Triphala Powder if not allergic to dairy. Others can have Triphala powder in warm water.

-Mediate for 10-15 minutes.

-Do the Breathing Techniques to be done before going to bed.

Chapter 20: Chart For Days 8-14

Days: 8-12

-Start your day with the Breathing Techniques to be done on waking up.

-Meditate for 20 minutes.

-Do the Breathing Techniques to be done on standing up.

-Have FRESH grape juice (black) without ice or sugar. Do not refrigerate. Have at room temperature.

-Have few strawberries or some soft fruit and a handful of almonds.

-Start moving. Go for a walk or do some mild exercises for 40 minutes.

-Get exposure to sunlight for 30 minutes.

-Have a breakfast high in protein, complex carbohydrates and fiber within 2 hours of waking up.

-Have a light nutritious meal with plenty of veggies and yogurt.

-Have 2 freshly made pita bread or Indian bread or rice with vegetables for dinner.

-Apply the Neem oil or Neem paste all over the body and relax for an hour before washing off with a mild soap. If Neem powder or paste was used instead of oil, there is no need for soap. This ought to be done in the day time between 7am and 4 pm.

-Before going to bed have warm organic Milk with Triphala Powder if not allergic to dairy. Others can have Triphala powder in warm water.

-Mediate for 20 minutes.

-Do the Breathing Techniques to be done before going to bed.

Day: 13

-Start your day with the Breathing Techniques to be done on waking up.

-Meditate for 30 minutes.

-Do the Breathing Techniques to be done on standing up.

-Have FRESH Pomegranate juice without ice or sugar. Do not refrigerate. Have at room temperature.

-Fast until 3 pm

-During fasting the patient can have fresh juice of apple, pomegranate, grapes and watermelon once in an hour. Do not refrigerate the juice. Do not add ice or sugar. Make fresh juice right before drinking.

-At 3pm, have a very light nutritious meal with veggies and yogurt.

Have a full body MASSAGE from your spouse or your therapist. Or have a self-massage done. And finish with a nice hot bath. Do not spend more than 20 minutes in the bath.

-Herbal wrap need not be done on the days of fasting.

-For dinner have 2 freshly made pita bread or Indian bread or rice with vegetables for dinner. This will be the only solid meal of the day and must be finished before 7 pm.

-Before going to bed have warm organic Milk with Triphala Powder if not allergic to dairy. Others can have Triphala powder in warm water.

-Mediate for 30 minutes.

-Do the Breathing Techniques to be done before going to bed.

Day 14

-Start your day early with the Breathing Techniques to be done on waking up.

-Meditate for 30 minutes.

-Do the Breathing Techniques to be done on standing up.

-Fast until afternoon. Stay indoors. Turn off TV, music and phones on this day.

-During fasting, drink cool water. Remember to never gulp down the water but sip and drink your water very slowly.

-Spread a cotton sheet on the floor and lie down on it. Keep your eyes closed and your mind clear. Try to have happy, peaceful, positive thoughts.

-If you feel too tired to fast with just water, you can have a glass of pomegranate

juice or honey in warm water once in an hour to keep up your energy levels. This can be taken until 11 am. Stop all kinds of juices at 11 am. A glass of water an hour is mandatory though.

-Around 1 pm, consume 5 tablespoons full of Neem oil. Drink a glass of hot water. Lie down flat on your back. Breathe deeply and slowly.

-The detox begins in 2 hours. The patient will feel nauseous. Vomiting and loose stools are normal part of detox. There is nothing to worry.

-Try to have Oral Rehydration Salts (ORS) every 30 minutes. You can buy a good brand of Oral Rehydration Salts from the pharmacist and mix with water instead of buying the ORS in drink form (to avoid the preservatives). Or mix 3 pinches of

sugar with 3 pinches of salt in a glass of water to make your homemade rehydration drink.

-After every single vomiting or toilet session, have few sips of your rehydration drink.

-If you don't start vomiting or pass loose stools or experience nausea within 90 minutes of having the Neem Oil, try to take another dose of 5 Tablespoons full of Neem Oil.

-Once it is all over, have a warm bath. Do not stay in the bath for more than 10 minutes.

-Have 2 freshly made pita bread or Indian bread or rice with vegetables for dinner.

-Before going to bed have warm organic Milk with Triphala Powder if not allergic to dairy. Others can have Triphala powder in warm water.

-Mediate for 30 minutes.

-Do the Breathing Techniques to be done before going to bed.

Chapter 21: Chart For Days 15-21

Days: 15-19

-Start your day with the Breathing Techniques to be done on waking up.

-Meditate for 30 minutes.

-Do the Breathing Techniques to be done on standing up.

-Have a glass of warm water with 1 teaspoon of honey and half a lemon.

-Have a serving of fruit and a handful of almonds.

-Start moving. Go for a walk or do some mild exercises for 40 minutes.

-Get exposure to sunlight for 30 minutes.

-Have a breakfast high in protein, complex carbohydrates and fiber within 2 hours of waking up.

-Have a light nutritious meal with plenty of veggies and yogurt.

-Can have 2 freshly made pita bread or Indian bread or rice with vegetables for dinner.

-Apply the Olive leaf paste all over the body and relax for an hour before washing off with a mild soap. If fresh Olive leaves are not available, you can use dry powder. Mix the dry powder in hot water and let it sit undisturbed for 30 minutes.

This ought to be done in the day time between 7am and 4 pm.

-Before going to bed have warm organic Milk with Triphala Powder if not allergic to dairy. Others can have Triphala powder in warm water.

-Mediate for 30 minutes.

-Do the Breathing Techniques to be done before going to bed.

Day: 20

-Start your day with the Breathing Techniques to be done on waking up.

-Meditate for 30 minutes.

-Do the Breathing Techniques to be done on standing up.

-Have FRESH Pomegranate juice without ice or sugar. Do not refrigerate. Have at room temperature.

-Fast until 3 pm

-During fasting the patient can have fresh juice of apple, pomegranate, grapes and watermelon once in an hour. Do not refrigerate the juice. Do not add ice or sugar. Make fresh juice right before drinking.

-At 3pm, have a very light nutritious meal with veggies and yogurt.

-Have a full body MASSAGE from your spouse or your therapist. Or have a self-massage done. And finish with a nice hot bath. Do not spend more than 20 minutes in the bath.

-Herbal wrap need not be done on the days of fasting.

For dinner have 2 freshly made pita bread or Indian bread or rice with vegetables for dinner. This will be the only solid meal of the day and must be finished before 7 pm.

-Before going to bed have warm organic Milk with Triphala Powder if not allergic to dairy. Others can have Triphala powder in warm water.

-Mediate for 30 minutes.

-Do the Breathing Techniques to be done before going to bed.

Day 21

-Start your day early with the Breathing Techniques to be done on waking up.

-Meditate for 40 minutes.

-Do the Breathing Techniques to be done on standing up.

-Fast until afternoon. Stay indoors. Turn off TV, music and phones on this day.

-During fasting, drink cool water. Remember to never gulp down the water but sip and drink your water very slowly.

-Spread a cotton sheet on the floor and lie down on it. Keep your eyes closed and your mind clear. Try to have happy, peaceful, positive thoughts.

-If you feel too tired to fast with just water, you can have a glass of pomegranate juice or honey in warm water once in an hour to keep up your energy levels. This can be taken until 11 am. Stop all kinds of juices at 11 am. A glass of water an hour is mandatory.

-Around 6 am, consume 3 tablespoons full of Castor Oil. Drink a glass of hot water after consuming the same. Lie down flat on your back. Breathe deeply and slowly.

-Have 3 tablespoons full of Neem Oil after an hour.

-The effective detox begins in 2 hours of taking Neem Oil but the Castor Oil will start the colon cleansing even before that. The patient will feel nauseous. Vomiting and loose stools are normal part of detox. There is nothing to worry.

-Try to have Oral Rehydration Salts (ORS) every 30 minutes. You can buy a good brand of Oral Rehydration Salts from the pharmacist and mix with water instead of buying the ORS in drink form (to avoid the preservatives). Or mix 3 pinches of

sugar with 3 pinches of salt in a glass of water to make your homemade rehydration drink.

-After every single vomiting or toilet session, have few sips of your rehydration drink.

-If you don't start vomiting or pass loose stools or experience nausea within 90 minutes of having the Neem Oil, try to take another dose of 3 Tablespoons full of Neem Oil.

-Once it is all over, have a warm bath. Do not stay in the bath for more than 10 minutes.

-Have 2 freshly made pita bread or Indian bread or rice with vegetables for dinner.

-Before going to bed have warm organic Milk with Triphala Powder if not allergic to dairy. Others can have Triphala powder in warm water.

-Mediate for 30 minutes. If you are too tired or sleepy, just meditate for 10 minutes and go to bed.

-Do the Breathing Techniques to be done before going to bed.

Chapter 22: Chart For Days 22-28

Days 22-26

-Start your day with the Breathing Techniques to be done on waking up.

-Meditate for 30 minutes.

-Do the Breathing Techniques to be done on standing up.

-Have a huge glass of warm water with 1 teaspoon of honey and a FULL lemon.

-Have a serving of fruit and a handful of almonds.

-Start moving. Go for a walk or do some mild exercises for 40 minutes.

-Get exposure to sunlight for 30 minutes.

-Have a breakfast high in protein, complex carbohydrates and fiber within 2 hours of waking up.

-Have a light nutritious meal with plenty of veggies and yogurt.

-Can have 2 freshly made pita bread or Indian bread or rice with vegetables for dinner.

-Apply the Neem Oil all over the body and relax for an hour before washing off with a mild soap. If possible try to do it between 7 am and 8 am and lay there in the sunlight (wearing a thin cotton garment) for an hour before having a hot bath. This ought to be done in the day time between 7am and 4 pm (preferably between 7 am and 8 am).

-Before going to bed have warm organic Milk with Triphala Powder if not allergic to dairy. Others can have Triphala powder in warm water.

-Mediate for 30 minutes.

-Do the Breathing Techniques to be done before going to bed.

Day: 27

-Start your day with the Breathing Techniques to be done on waking up.

-Meditate for 30 minutes.

-Do the Breathing Techniques to be done on standing up.

- Have a glass of raw papaya smoothie without ice or sugar. Do not refrigerate. Have at room temperature. Add a spoonful of pumpkin seeds to the smoothie.

- Fast until 3 pm

- During fasting the patient can have fresh juice of apple, pomegranate, grapes and watermelon once in an hour. Do not refrigerate the juice. Do not add ice or sugar. Make fresh juice right before drinking.

- At 3pm, have a very light nutritious meal with veggies and yogurt.

- Have a full body MASSAGE from your spouse or your therapist. Or have a self-massage done. And finish with a nice hot bath. Do not spend more than 20 minutes in the bath.

-Herbal wrap need not be done on the days of fasting.

-For dinner have 2 freshly made pita bread or Indian bread or rice with vegetables for dinner. This will be the only solid meal of the day and must be finished before 7 pm.

-Before going to bed have warm organic Milk with Triphala Powder if not allergic to dairy. Others can have Triphala powder in warm water.

-Mediate for 30 minutes.

-Do the Breathing Techniques to be done before going to bed.

Day 21

-Start your day early with the Breathing Techniques to be done on waking up.

-Meditate for 40 minutes.

-Do the Breathing Techniques to be done on standing up.

-Fast until afternoon. Stay indoors. Turn off TV, music and phones on this day.

-During fasting, drink cool water. Remember to never gulp down the water but sip and drink your water very slowly.

-Spread a cotton sheet on the floor and lie down on it. Keep your eyes closed and your mind clear. Try to have happy, peaceful, positive thoughts.

-If you feel too tired to fast with just water, you can have a glass of pomegranate

juice or honey in warm water once in an hour to keep up your energy levels. This can be taken until 11 am. Stop all kinds of juices at 11 am. A glass of water an hour is mandatory.

-Around 6 am, consume 50 grams of fresh Neem Paste. Have a glass of water after swallowing the paste. To swallow it fast, swish around a tablespoon of Olive Oil in your mouth and

-If you cannot get fresh Neem paste, try to get dry Neem leaves or dry Neem leaves powder and make a decoction of it (by adding 50 grams of it to the boiling water of 3 glasses). Drink after it gets warm. Lie down flat on your back. Breathe deeply and slowly.

-The patient will feel nauseous. Vomiting and loose stools are normal part of detox. There is nothing to worry.

-Try to have Oral Rehydration Salts (ORS) every 30 minutes. You can buy a good brand of Oral Rehydration Salts from the pharmacist and mix with water instead of buying the ORS in drink form (to avoid the preservatives). Or mix 3 pinches of sugar with 3 pinches of salt in a glass of water to make your homemade rehydration drink.

-After every single vomiting or toilet session, have few sips of your rehydration drink.

-If you don't start vomiting or pass loose stools or experience nausea within 90 minutes of having the Neem Oil, try to take a dose of 3 Tablespoons full of Neem Oil.

-Once it is all over, have a warm bath. Do not stay in the bath for more than 10 minutes.

-Have 2 freshly made pita bread or Indian bread or rice with vegetables for dinner.

-Before going to bed have warm organic Milk with Triphala Powder if not allergic to dairy. Others can have Triphala powder in warm water.

-Mediate for 30 minutes. If you are too tired or sleepy, just meditate for 10 minutes and go to bed.

-Do the Breathing Techniques to be done before going to bed.

Chapter 23: Chart For Days 29-35

Days: 29-33

-Start your day with the Breathing Techniques to be done on waking up.

-Meditate for 30 minutes.

-Do the Breathing Techniques to be done on standing up.

-Have a glass of this juice made from carrot-beet-apple-juice (in the ratio of 1:0.5:1 with a teaspoon of honey).

-Have a serving of fruit and a handful of almonds.

-Start moving. Go for a walk or do some mild exercises for 40 minutes.

-Get exposure to sunlight for 30 minutes.

-Have a breakfast high in protein, complex carbohydrates and fiber within 2 hours of waking up.

-Have a light nutritious meal with plenty of veggies and yogurt.

-Can have 2 freshly made pita bread or Indian bread or rice with vegetables for dinner.

-Apply a mixture of Castor Oil and Neem Oil (in equal quantities) all over the body and relax for an hour before washing off with a mild soap. This ought to be done in the day time between 7am and 4 pm.

-Before going to bed have warm organic Milk with Triphala Powder if not allergic to dairy. Others can have Triphala powder in warm water.

-Mediate for 30 minutes.

-Do the Breathing Techniques to be done before going to bed.

Day: 34

-Start your day with the Breathing Techniques to be done on waking up.

-Meditate for 30 minutes.

-Do the Breathing Techniques to be done on standing up.

-Have FRESH Pomegranate juice without ice or sugar. Do not refrigerate. Have at room temperature.

-Fast until 3 pm

-During fasting the patient can have fresh juice of apple, pomegranate, grapes and watermelon once in an hour. Do not refrigerate the juice. Do not add ice or sugar. Make fresh juice right before drinking.

-At 3pm, have a very light nutritious meal with veggies and yogurt.

-Have a full body MASSAGE from your spouse or your therapist. Or have a self-massage done. And finish with a nice hot bath. Do not spend more than 20 minutes in the bath.

-Herbal wrap need not be done on the days of fasting.

-For dinner have 2 freshly made pita bread or Indian bread or rice with vegetables for dinner. This will be the only solid meal of the day and must be finished before 7 pm.

−Before going to bed have warm organic Milk with Triphala Powder if not allergic to dairy. Others can have Triphala powder in warm water.

−Mediate for 30 minutes.

−Do the Breathing Techniques to be done before going to bed.

Day 35

−Start your day early with the Breathing Techniques to be done on waking up.

−Meditate for 40 minutes.

-Do the Breathing Techniques to be done on standing up.

-Fast until afternoon. Stay indoors. Turn off TV, music and phones on this day.

-During fasting, drink cool water. Remember to never gulp down the water but sip and drink your water very slowly.

-Spread a cotton sheet on the floor and lie down on it. Keep your eyes closed and your mind clear. Try to have happy, peaceful, positive thoughts.

-Strict water fasting.

-Around 6 am, consume 3 tablespoons full of Castor Oil. Drink a glass of hot water after consuming the same. Lie down flat on your back. Breathe deeply and slowly.

-Have 3 tablespoons full of Neem Oil after an hour of consuming the Castor Oil.

-The effective detox begins in 2 hours of taking Neem Oil. The patient will feel nauseous. Vomiting and loose stools are normal part of detox. There is nothing to worry.

-Try to have Oral Rehydration Salts (ORS) every 30 minutes. You can buy a good brand of Oral Rehydration Salts from the pharmacist and mix with water instead of buying the ORS in drink form (to avoid the preservatives). Or mix 3 pinches of sugar with 3 pinches of salt in a glass of water to make your homemade rehydration drink.

-After every single vomiting or toilet session, have few sips of your rehydration drink.

-If you don't start vomiting or pass loose stools or experience nausea within 90 minutes of having the Neem Oil, try to take another dose of 3 Tablespoons full of Neem Oil.

-Once it is all over, have a warm bath. Do not stay in the bath for more than 10 minutes.

-Have 2 freshly made pita bread or Indian bread or rice with vegetables for dinner.

-Before going to bed have warm organic Milk with Triphala Powder if not allergic to dairy. Others can have Triphala powder in warm water.

-Mediate for 30 minutes. If you are too tired or sleepy, just meditate for 10 minutes and go to bed.

–Do the Breathing Techniques to be done before going to bed.

Chapter 24: Chart For Days 36-42

Days: 36-40

-Start your day with the Breathing Techniques to be done on waking up.

-Meditate for 30 minutes.

-Do the Breathing Techniques to be done on standing up.

-Have a glass of warm water with 1 teaspoon of honey and a FULL lemon.

-Have a serving of fruit and a handful of almonds.

-Start moving. Go for a walk or do some mild exercises for 40 minutes.

-Get exposure to sunlight for 30 minutes.

-Have a breakfast high in protein, complex carbohydrates and fiber within 2 hours of waking up.

-Have a light nutritious meal with plenty of veggies and yogurt.

-Can have 2 freshly made pita bread or Indian bread or rice with vegetables for dinner.

-Mix turmeric powder in Olive Oil and apply all over the body. Let it stay for an hour. Wash off with warm water. This ought to be done in the day time between 7am and 4 pm.

-Before going to bed have warm organic Milk with Triphala Powder if not allergic to dairy. Others can have Triphala powder in warm water.

-Mediate for 30 minutes.

-Do the Breathing Techniques to be done before going to bed.

Day: 41

-Start your day with the Breathing Techniques to be done on waking up.

-Meditate for 30 minutes.

-Do the Breathing Techniques to be done on standing up.

-Have FRESH Pomegranate juice without ice or sugar. Do not refrigerate. Have at room temperature.

- Fast until 3 pm

- During fasting the patient can have fresh juice of apple, pomegranate, grapes and watermelon once in an hour. Do not refrigerate the juice. Do not add ice or sugar. Make fresh juice right before drinking.

- At 3pm, have a very light nutritious meal with veggies and yogurt.

- Have a full body MASSAGE from your spouse or your therapist. Or have a self-massage done. And finish with a nice hot bath. Do not spend more than 20 minutes in the bath.

- Herbal wrap (Neem, Aloe, Olive, etc.) need not be done on the days of fasting.

-For dinner have 2 freshly made pita bread or Indian bread or rice with vegetables for dinner. This will be the only solid meal of the day and must be finished before 7 pm.

-Before going to bed have warm organic Milk with Triphala Powder if not allergic to dairy. Others can have Triphala powder in warm water.

-Mediate for 30 minutes.

-Do the Breathing Techniques to be done before going to bed.

Day: 42

-Start your day early with the Breathing Techniques to be done on waking up.

-Meditate for 40 minutes.

-Do the Breathing Techniques to be done on standing up.

-Fast until afternoon. Stay indoors. Turn off TV, music and phones on this day.

-During fasting, drink cool water. Remember to never gulp down the water but sip and drink your water very slowly.

-Spread a cotton sheet on the floor and lie down on it. Keep your eyes closed and your mind clear. Try to have happy, peaceful, positive thoughts.

-Strict fasting. Only water can be consumed.

-Around 6 am, consume 3 tablespoons full of Neem Oil. Drink a glass of hot water after consuming the same. Lie down flat on your back. Breathe deeply and slowly.

-Have 3 tablespoons full of Neem Oil again after an hour of taking the Neem Oil.

-The effective detox begins in 2 hours of taking Neem Oil. The patient will feel nauseous. Vomiting and loose stools are normal part of detox. There is nothing to worry.

-Try to have Oral Rehydration Salts (ORS) every 30 minutes. You can buy a good brand of Oral Rehydration Salts from the pharmacist and mix with water instead of buying the ORS in drink form (to avoid the preservatives). Or mix 3 pinches of sugar with 3 pinches of salt in a glass of water to make your homemade rehydration drink.

-After every single vomiting or toilet session, have few sips of your rehydration drink.

-Once it is all over, have a warm bath. Do not stay in the bath for more than 10 minutes.

-Have 2 freshly made pita bread or Indian bread or rice with vegetables for dinner.

-Before going to bed have warm organic Milk with Triphala Powder if not allergic to dairy. Others can have Triphala powder in warm water.

-Mediate for 30 minutes. If you are too tired or sleepy, just meditate for 10 minutes and go to bed.

-Do the Breathing Techniques to be done before going to bed.

Chapter 24: Chart For Days 36-42

Chapter 25: Chart For Days 43-49

Days: 43-47

-Start your day with the Breathing Techniques to be done on waking up.

-Meditate for 30 minutes.

-Do the Breathing Techniques to be done on standing up.

-Have a glass of warm water with 1 teaspoon of honey and half a lemon.

-Have a serving of fruit and a handful of almonds.

-Start moving. Go for a walk or do some mild exercises for 40 minutes.

-Get exposure to sunlight for 30 minutes.

-Have a breakfast high in protein, complex carbohydrates and fiber within 2 hours of waking up.

-Have a light nutritious meal with plenty of veggies and yogurt.

-Can have 2 freshly made pita bread or Indian bread or rice with vegetables for dinner.

-Apply the Olive leaf paste all over the body and relax for an hour before washing off with a mild soap. If fresh Olive leaves are not available, you can use dry powder. Mix the dry powder in hot water and let it sit undisturbed for 30 minutes. Or use Neem Leaf Powder or fresh Neem Paste. This ought to be done in the day time between 7am and 4 pm. Best time is between 7am to 8am.

-Before going to bed have warm organic Milk with Triphala Powder if not allergic to dairy. Others can have Triphala powder in warm water.

-Mediate for 30 minutes.

-Do the Breathing Techniques to be done before going to bed.

Day: 48

-Start your day with the Breathing Techniques to be done on waking up.

-Meditate for 30 minutes.

-Do the Breathing Techniques to be done on standing up.

-Have FRESH Pomegranate juice without ice or sugar. Do not refrigerate. Have at room temperature.

-Fast until 3 pm

-During fasting the patient can have fresh juice of apple, pomegranate, grapes and watermelon once in an hour. Do not refrigerate the juice. Do not add ice or sugar. Make fresh juice right before drinking.

-At 3pm, have a very light nutritious meal with veggies and yogurt.

-Have a full body MASSAGE from your spouse or your therapist. Or have a self-massage done. And finish with a nice hot bath. Do not spend more than 20 minutes in the bath.

-Herbal wrap of one hour need not be done on the days of fasting.

-For dinner have 2 freshly made pita bread or Indian bread or rice with vegetables for dinner. This will be the only solid meal of the day and must be finished before 7 pm.

-Before going to bed have warm organic Milk with Triphala Powder if not allergic to dairy. Others can have Triphala powder in warm water.

-Mediate for 30 minutes.

-Do the Breathing Techniques to be done before going to bed.

Day 49

-Start your day early with the Breathing Techniques to be done on waking up.

-Meditate for 40 minutes.

-Do the Breathing Techniques to be done on standing up.

-Fast until afternoon. Stay indoors. Turn off TV, music and phones on this day.

-During fasting, drink cool water. Remember to never gulp down the water but sip and drink your water very slowly.

-Spread a cotton sheet on the floor and lie down on it. Keep your eyes closed and your mind clear. Try to have happy, peaceful, positive thoughts.

-Strict fasting. Only water is allowed.

-Around 6 am, consume 5 tablespoons full of Neem Oil. Lie down flat on your back. Breathe deeply and slowly.

-The patient will feel nauseous. Vomiting and loose stools are normal part of detox. There is nothing to worry.

-Try to have Oral Rehydration Salts (ORS) every 30 minutes. You can buy a good brand of Oral Rehydration Salts from the pharmacist and mix with water instead of buying the ORS in drink form (to avoid the preservatives). Or mix 3 pinches of sugar with 3 pinches of salt in a glass of water to make your homemade rehydration drink.

-After every single vomiting or toilet session, have few sips of your rehydration drink.

-If you don't start vomiting or pass loose stools or experience nausea within 90 minutes of having the Neem Oil, try to take another dose of 3 Tablespoons full of Neem Oil.

-Once it is all over, have a warm bath. Do not stay in the bath for more than 10 minutes.

-Have 2 freshly made pita bread or Indian bread or rice with vegetables for dinner.

-Before going to bed have warm organic Milk with Triphala Powder if not allergic to dairy. Others can have Triphala powder in warm water.

–Mediate for 30 minutes. If you are too tired or sleepy, just meditate for 10 minutes and go to bed.

–Do the Breathing Techniques to be done before going to bed.

Chapter 26: Chart For Days 50, 51 and 52.

-Start your day early with the Breathing Techniques to be done on waking up.

-Meditate for 40 minutes.

-Do the Breathing Techniques to be done on standing up.

-Fast until afternoon. Stay indoors. Turn off TV, music and phones on this day.

-During fasting, drink cool water. Remember to never gulp down the water but sip and drink your water very slowly.

–Spread a cotton sheet on the floor and lie down on it. Keep your eyes closed and your mind clear. Try to have happy, peaceful, positive thoughts.

–Strict fasting. Only water is allowed.

–Around 6 am, consume 7 tablespoons full of Neem Oil. Lie down flat on your back. Breathe deeply and slowly.

–The patient will feel nauseous. Vomiting and loose stools are normal part of detox. There is nothing to worry.

–Try to have Oral Rehydration Salts (ORS) every 30 minutes. You can buy a good brand of Oral Rehydration Salts from the pharmacist and mix with water instead of buying the ORS in drink form (to avoid the preservatives). Or mix 3 pinches of sugar with 3 pinches of salt in a glass of water to make your homemade rehydration drink.

-After every single vomiting or toilet session, have few sips of your rehydration drink.

-If you don't start vomiting or pass loose stools or experience nausea within 90 minutes of having the Neem Oil, try to take another dose of 3 Tablespoons full of Neem Oil.

-Once it is all over, have a warm bath. Do not stay in the bath for more than 10 minutes.

-Have 2 freshly made pita bread or Indian bread or rice with vegetables for dinner.

-Before going to bed have warm organic Milk with Triphala Powder if not allergic to dairy. Others can have Triphala powder in warm water.

—Mediate for 30 minutes. If you are too tired or sleepy, just meditate for 10 minutes and go to bed.

—Do the Breathing Techniques to be done before going to bed.

Dear reader, you will start feeling much better by the 52nd day. If necessary, repeat the whole process again after an interval of 2 months.

Note: 50 grams of Olive Leaves Extract can be used on the 7th Detox day of every 7 day cycle along with regular detox.

Before We Part

Dear Reader

As I started contemplating about this project a few months ago, many people got quite concerned on so many levels. It was not just against their religious beliefs but their personal beliefs & values too. True Christians have genuine love for others while the fake Christians love to condemn others and mock them, to feel better about themselves.

I was pestered with questions. Am I going to help those horny sex-addicts and hookers with this book? Am I going to assure the adulterous men and women to go ahead and sin without worrying about the drastic consequences? Religious people often assume that everybody else is a worst sinner than they are.

They opined that it was wrong on my part to inform the world about the natural solution for sexually transmitted diseases while it is clearly a punishment for sins! (I am sure this might be offensive but stay with me for the rest of the journey.) While most of the diseases are punishments for the sins we have committed knowingly or unknowingly, or the painful consequences of deliberate negligence and carelessness (sins caused by not doing what we ought to do), or something we undergo for some good, Jesus clearly stated that it is not God's will that any of us shall perish.

WHO IS FREE OF SIN? GOD LOVES US ANYWAY!

And again, Jesus came not for the self-righteous but for the sinners! Bible says that every single one of us have sinned in one way or the other and have fallen short of glory. 1John1 ends with a verse which declares that anyone who claims that he/she hasn't sinned is a liar, and is calling God a liar, for God says that we have sinned.

It is for the same reason that I never talk about the reversal of ageing with anyone unless I know them personally and I am convinced that they wouldn't become a stumbling block to others. Many experts in alternate medicine knows such techniques but refuses to impart knowledge in fear that it will end in the hands of wrong people who are better off dead. I, personally, cannot forgive myself if my book helps a bad person to live stronger and healthy.... a person who would make life difficult for others, say, a murderer or a pedophile or a rapist.

I sat there in my study and constantly reflected on this matter in my prayers; I was assured by The Holy Spirit that I can go ahead with this project. I am going against the self-righteous Pharisees of today in making this 'controversial' book available to the general public.

Those people who are affected with sexually transmitted diseases are not criminals. Not everyone with herpes is a hooker, sex-addict or pedophile. But then, God loves even them (hookers, etc.) for Jesus died for the sinners! Who are we to judge? They are humans loved by God, and I love them because they are loved by God. I do pray that it doesn't help the bad people who might harm others.

Getting healed naturally requires a great deal of discipline and determination! I pray that you find the discipline and determination to follow what I say here, and thereby change your life for the better–forever.

I hope my book helps the right kind of people who wouldn't be a danger to anyone. I pray God's peace and love over you and your loved ones who read this book. May God, The Almighty greatly bless you and grant you good health.

Take care for you truly deserve it. Deserving because God loves you no matter what anyone else claims. Nothing is as satisfying as having a good health! God bless you.

–Richard T. Frank

About the author

Richard Teddy Frank is the pen name of the author who is an accountant by profession and a wellness expert by passion. He paints and writes when he gets leisure time.

Helping people to treat their diseases and medical conditions by bringing awareness about the many natural cures available is one of the primary goals of the author.

Your Notes

Kindly try to put into action what you read here. Buying books and medicines won't cure the disease. Using them is important.

www.ingramcontent.com/pod-product-compliance
Lightning Source LLC
Chambersburg PA
CBHW021429170526
45164CB00001B/157